TABLE OF CONTENTS

INTRODUCTION

As someone interested in the world of keto, you've likely heard (or read) about its incredible potential for weight loss, mental sharpness, and more! A well designed ketogenic diet is a virtually unmatched tool for managing your weight (and many chronic health conditions) as well as supporting your cognitive acuity and overall healthy aging regimen.

With the exploding popularity of the keto diet, you'll undoubtedly find countless approaches and tips out there, focusing only on increasing fat consumption or avoiding carbohydrates at any cost. In my experience, these strategies miss the bigger picture of what keto should be—and what is possible with the keto diet.

The ketogenic diet is often regarded as a brutal regimen to follow; however, with practice, and an understanding of what the diet aims to achieve, it can be reduced to a manageable routine. The basic aim is to switch the body's primary fuel source from carbohydrates (like bread and sugar) to fats. This is done by increasing the intake of fats and significantly reducing the intake of carbohydrates. The real difficulty is that the diet is so restrictive that all foods eaten must be weighed out to a tenth of a gram during meal preparation, and a participant may not eat anything which is not "prescribed" by the dietician. The level of carbohydrates allowed is shallow, so that even the small amount of sugar in most liquid or chewable medications will prevent the diet from working.

For example, a typical meal might include some meat with green vegetables cooked with a mayonnaise sauce or a lot of butter. Heavy cream may be included on the side for drinking. Another meal might consist of bacon and eggs with many butters or oil added and heavy cream to drink. A very high ratio of fats to carbohydrates must be maintained with a low total calorie intake for the diet to be successful.

KETO

As someone interested in the world of keto, you've likely heard (or read) about its incredible potential for weight loss, mental sharpness, and more! A well designed ketogenic diet is a virtually unmatched tool for managing your weight (and many chronic health conditions) as well as supporting your cognitive acuity and overall healthy aging regimen.

With the exploding popularity of the keto diet, you'll undoubtedly find countless approaches and tips out there, focusing only on increasing fat consumption or avoiding carbohydrates at any cost. In my experience, these strategies miss the bigger picture of what keto should be—and what is possible with the keto diet.

The ketogenic diet is often regarded as a brutal regimen to follow; however, with practice, and an understanding of what the diet aims to achieve, it can be reduced to a manageable routine. The basic aim is to switch the body's primary fuel source from carbohydrates (like bread and sugar) to fats. This is done by increasing the intake of fats and significantly reducing the intake of carbohydrates. The real difficulty is that the diet is so restrictive that all foods eaten must be weighed out to a tenth of a gram during meal preparation, and a participant may not eat anything which is not "prescribed" by the dietician. The level of carbohydrates allowed is shallow, so that even the small amount of sugar in most liquid or chewable medications will prevent the diet from working.

For example, a typical meal might include some meat with green vegetables cooked with a mayonnaise sauce or a lot of butter. Heavy cream may be included on the side for drinking. Another meal might consist of bacon and eggs with many butters or oil added and heavy cream to drink. A very high ratio of fats to carbohydrates must be maintained with a low total calorie intake for the diet to be successful.

WHAT IS KETOGENIC DIET?

A Ketogenic Diet is any diet that causes ketones to be produced by the liver, shifting the body's metabolism away from glucose towards fat utilization. Typically on a moderate to high carb diet, the body will prefer glucose for fuel (usually from dietary carbs), but by restricting carbs, the body will prefer fat for fuel. By inducing ketosis, a series of adaptations will take place.

Ketosis is also an effective way to control your blood sugar. When you eat something high in carbohydrates, your body produces insulin to get rid of all the sugar in your blood. But since there are already carbs to be used for fuel, your body will be storing fat cells and not releasing any to be burned. So by reducing carbs and being in ketosis, your insulin levels will be regulated at a lower level, and your body will want to access your body fat for fuel instead. In most cases, this means impressive weight-loss!

With controlled blood sugar levels, you will experience less hunger and cravings. Paired with an adequate protein and high fat intake, you will feel both satisfied and satiated by the diet. What do I eat?

A typical Ketogenic Diet is any diet that restricts carbohydrates between 0- 50g of carbs per day. The general recommendation of keto is to start with 20g of net carbs per day. This limit does a good job of eliminating junk foods, refined carbohydrates, and any other "fattening" foods.

Net carbs are the total carbs minus the fiber carbs (fiber doesn't count because your body doesn't absorb it). For example, a cup of chopped broccoli is 6g of total carbs and 2g of fiber. 6g - 2g = 4g net carbs.

Your carbs should ideally come from whole-food sources such as vegetables, nuts, dairy, etc. Try your best to avoid refined carbohydrates such as bread, pasta, and cereals; starches such as potatoes, beans, and legumes; and other refined sugars such as white sugar, HFCS, and even sugar from fruits.

Most meals should focus on protein and fat with a side of vegetables. Some examples would be; a steak with a side of sautéed spinach or chicken thighs with a side of broccoli and cheese sauce. Snacks can include nuts and seeds, cheese, or anything "keto-friendly." When in doubt, check the nutrition label or google the carb count to see if it fits within your daily carb goal.

Side note: Be wary of claims such as 'effective carbs' or 'net carbs.' Many of these items will use sugar alcohols, which do in-fact count (at least partially) and will have an effect on your blood sugar.

Adequate protein is also a very important aspect of the Ketogenic Diet, and it will help you preserve muscle mass.

What portion of fat/protein/carbs do I need?

One of the mantras of low-carb diets is the ratio of macronutrients "60/35/5". This means that the percentage of your daily caloric intake needs to be sixty percent from fat, thirty-five from protein, and five from carbohydrates. Fat and protein keep you full, so more of them are often preferred to naturally keep you in a calorie deficit. Though macronutrient ratios are a good starting point, they aren't always accurate. Another method is to choose a carb goal between 15- 50g/day (20g is a good starting point), set your protein requirements (1.5-1.75g of protein per kilogram of ideal body weight), and fill the rest of your calories with fat.

Do I need to count calories?

In many cases, a Ketogenic Diet will help you reduce your caloric intake naturally. Some people don't count calories while others do, it's really a personal decision! But if you aren't counting calories and you find your weight-loss is stalling, then consider tracking.

What happens when my body adapts?

You may experience nausea, headaches, dizziness, mental fog, and other flu- like symptoms. This phenomenon is often called 'keto-flu' or 'carb-flu. Many times this is the result of your electrolytes being flushed out along with water weight. If you drink some traditional chicken or beef broth, you can replenish your electrolytes and ease your symptoms. It is also incredibly important to drink plenty of water! Your water intake will keep you hydrated, and it will help flush out excess ketones.

Fun fact: The body can excrete up to 100 calories worth of ketones per day.

This total adaptation process takes about three weeks to happen. During this time, you may be continuing an exercise regimen, or you may even be starting a new one. You may find that you don't have as much endurance and strength as you are used to, and this is normal. Once you are fully keto-adapted, your body will be trained to operate on fat as its primary source of fuel, and you will see an improvement in your energy levels. Many even report having more energy and more stable energy levels while in ketosis.

How do I guarantee I'm in ketosis?

An easy way to know for sure you are in ketosis is to use ketosis. These little sticks can be found in most pharmacies and even online. They only test for excess ketones, so they aren't always the most reliable, but if you see a positive on the stick, you are guaranteed to be in ketosis. Other signs of ketosis might be; a funny taste in your mouth, your urine will smell different, or you're incredibly thirsty. But if you have been eating 20g of carbs a day for at least 3 days, you are more than likely in ketosis.

I don't think I can give up carbs!

Once you get over the initial hump of carb cravings, they go away! Since keto will stabilize your blood sugar, it will also stabilize your hunger and cravings. Since your body is now adjusting to a low-sugar diet, you will find that your

taste buds will change as well, and you can now easily detect the sugar content in certain foods. Items such as carrots and dark chocolate now taste sweeter. The longer you stick to keto and the stricter you are, the less you will miss carbs. Carbs and sugar are truly addictive, and like anyone else trying to break an addiction, the best method is to cut out the source of the problem.

What is the Keto Reset Diet?

The Keto Reset Diet is a particular approach to keto that prioritizes nutrient density and natural, whole food eating. It's the approach I live (and promote) because it's a sustainable means of achieving and maintaining ketosis without compromising overall nutrition or health.

In other words, you get all the metabolic advantages of ketosis (lower insulin levels, lower inflammation, more" even" energy and cognitive function, etc.) And the critical benefits of a nutrient-dense diet. With the general suggestion of 50 grams of carbs per day, the Keto Reset Diet offers a generous window to enjoy a flavorful, varied diet every day.

HOW DOES THE KETOGENIC DIET WORK?

The food we eat provides the fuel used by our bodies for everyday activities and the materials needed to help the body grow. Unlike cars, which can only run on gasoline, the body is designed o use three primary fuels, including carbohydrates, fats, and protein. Carbohydrates are the primary component of sugars, starch, and flour, which come mostly from plants. Fats come in two broad types: saturated fats, like butter, which mostly come from animals, and unsaturated fats, like corn oil, which mostly come from plants. Finally, protein comes mainly from animals and is represented by meat and fish.

The preceding is a broad generalization, and there are many variations, such as nuts, which contain more than 50% fat. Carbohydrates, fats, and proteins all undergo the same type of chemical reaction with the oxygen we breathe to produce energy for the body, and waste products, including carbon dioxide and water, is the same reaction seen when a car engine burns gasoline or when wood or coal e burned for heat, etc. Although all three of the body's fuels are metabolized in the same way, carbohydrates are used preferentially, followed by fats than proteins.

Carbohydrates are used preferentially because they are usually readily available in most people, and the body can metabolize them quickly for energy. Athletes often eat some form of high-carbohydrate snacks before an athletic event to provide extra energy.

Typically carbohydrates will be used within a few hours after they are eaten, which is why we eat so frequently. Unused carbohydrates are stored in the liver in the form of glycogen or converted to fat.

In contrast, the primary role of fats is to store energy. Animals fatten up to prepare for winter. The body stores the fats we eat but, if there isn't enough carbohydrate available, the body will break down the fat stores to use as fuel. Fats are metabolized much more slowly, and typically it will take a day or so for the fat content of a meal to be used.

This is why people feel fuller after a fatty meal as opposed to a low carbohydrate meal. The third fuel, protein, is primarily used to build and replenish body materials; any excess protein is metabolized as fuel or excreted. If carbohydrate and fat stores are depleted, the body will begin to breakdown muscle to metabolize the protein for fuel.

In a typical western diet, the proportion (by weight) of the three fuels used will be about 5 – 15% protein, 10 – 20% fat, and 65 – 85 carbohydrate. Any excess "fuel" will be stored as fat by the body or excreted. By contrast, in the ketogenic diet, the proportion of fats is raised significantly, and the proportion of carbohydrates is greatly reduced.

It is also necessary to control the total intake of food Since if the body is given excess, it will discard the fats preferentially to get back to its preferred balance of fuels. By restricting the total caloric intake, the body is forced to metabolize fat in place of carbohydrates.

The ketogenic diet mimics a starvation or fasting state by denying the body the carbohydrate it requires to function normally and forcing it to metabolize fat. As the fat is metabolized, ketone bodies are produced. It is the production of the ketone bodies, which appears to play a central role in the ketogenic diet's success.

When the body begins producing ketone bodies, it is referred to as the body being in ketosis. It usually takes 3 – 5 days for the body to go into ketosis after starting the diet. Ketosis is readily recognized because the ketones can be detected in the urine and recognized by a characteristic smell of the individual's breath.

The ketogenic diet's prophylactic properties build up with time, and it may take several weeks before the full effect of the ketogenic diet is achieved.

Ketogenic Diet for Therapeutic Applications

Blood Lipids on a Ketogenic Diet: Lack of proper education has incorrectly held a high-fat diet responsible for increasing blood lipids. Decades of research, combined with efforts to shift the paradigm, reveal that increased dietary fat consumption does not directly result in increased blood lipids.

It is carbohydrate consumption that tends to increase total cholesterol with noticeable decreases in the HDL "good" cholesterol. Often, researchers use a "high-fat diet" interchangeably with a "Western diet;" many confuse the term "high-fat diet" in the research with a ketogenic diet. A "high-fat diet" in the research indicates a diet with high-fats and high-carbs, which is associated with increased blood lipids, whereas a ketogenic diet is not. For example, here are a couple of studies that have looked at this directly:

Consuming under 20g of carbohydrates/day compared to a low-fat, high- carbohydrate diet led to a 4x increase in HDL concentration.

A 12-week low carbohydrate diet led to a 10% decrease in LDL, a 5% increase in LDL particle size, and a 19% decrease in total VLDL particles (*Smaller LDL particle size is associated with a higher risk of developing atherosclerosis compared to larger LDL particles). Six months on a ketogenic diet led to an 11% decrease in LDL.

HOW DOES KETO WORK?

A ketogenic diet, or keto for short, is any diet that puts your body in a state of nutritional ketosis, and your body is burning fat (either body fat or fat that you eat) for fuel.

If you eat a high-carb diet (and most of us do), your body burns glucose for fuel. There are problems with glucose. The body can store about 2000 Calories of glucose energy at any one time in the form of glycogen. Once depleted, you can lose energy (sometimes called "bonking"), and you need sugar.

STAT! Excess glucose raises insulin. Insulin drives glucose into skeletal cells for storage as glycogen and burning. It also drives glucose into the liver for storage, glucose and burning, and conversion into fat. Glucose is also shipped out in LDL (or stored in the liver as foie gras). Insulin also drives glucose into fat cells to be converted into fat and stored. Fructose, one half of table sugar – and the sugar in all fruit, goes directly to the liver to be converted to fat. That's right. All fruit sugar, ½ of all table sugar, and high fructose corn syrup are NOT burned as energy. It's stored as fat.

Excess glucose in the blood can cause significant damage, as we've already discussed, leading to type 2 diabetes – a disease the medical establishment tells you is progressive, only gets worse, and cannot be reversed.

If you remove carbohydrates and instead eat moderate protein and higher fat levels, insulin levels drop because there is much less glucose to operate on. When insulin is low, your liver can burn fat for fuel. That's just the way it is. Your body can't burn stored fat unless insulin is low.

The byproduct of burning fat is ketones. Ketones are essential fatty acids that most cells in your body (including your brain, heart, and other organs) can use fuel directly. We are all born in nutritional ketosis. For 180,000 years, Homo Sapiens has been in nutritional ketosis most of the time, living on animal protein and fat – with rare plants, nuts, and fruits.

Just because your body is in ketosis doesn't mean that it's particularly good at using fat for fuel. It takes 3 to 8 weeks to become fully fat-adapted. Your body forgets how to deal with glucose effectively and instead gets very efficient at dealing with fat and the ketones that come from fat burning.

Once you are fully fat-adapted, you'll find you have an unending source of energy. You could run a marathon and not run out of juice. Your body fat is your new energy source, and it doesn't need to be replenished with food. Many advanced athletes are performing amazing feats of endurance while fasted! As long as the body can burn body fat, it's smooth sailing.

You can expect your cravings and hunger to disappear. As long as you stay away from carbs, you won't want them. The more fat-adapted you get, the less you'll want to eat "carbage." You can expect to return to a healthy body weight in a relatively short period.

What can I Eat on a Keto Diet?

- Meats – pork, poultry, fish, beef, lamb

- Eggs

- Leafy Greens – Spinach, kale,

- Vegetables that grow above – broccoli, cauliflower, cabbage, mushrooms

- High-fat dairy – butter, hard cheeses, high fat cream

- Nuts and seeds – macadamias, almonds, pecans, walnuts, sunflower seeds

- Avocado

- Berries- raspberries, blueberries,

- blackberries, etc.

- Sweeteners – stevia, allulose, erythritol, monk fruit, tagatose, inulin

- Other fats – coconut oil, high-fat salad dressing, saturated fats, etc.

Keto Macros & How to count them?

Getting to understand the macros according to your goals is essential to have great success on a keto diet. Protein is an essential macro that should you should always reach. Eating too little protein leads to muscle loss, and overeating protein can kick you out of ketosis. The fat intake depends on your goals. Not everyone is on the keto diet for weight loss. Some people are following the keto diet as a treatment/ control for different diseases. To find out the NET carbs, subtract the fiber and sugar alcohols (if in the product) from the TOTAL Carbs.

Vegetables on a Ketogenic Diet

Dark green and leafy is always the best choice for vegetables. Most of your meals should be protein with vegetables and an extra side of fat. Chicken

breast basted in olive oil, with broccoli and cheese. Steak topped with a knob of butter and a side of spinach sauteed in olive oil. If you're still confused about what a net carb is, don't worry – I'll explain further. Let's say, for example; you want to eat some broccoli (1 cup) – seriously, my favorite and most delicious vegetable out there.

- There are a total of 6g carbohydrates in 1 cup.

- There's also 2g of fiber in 1 cup.

- So, we take the 6g (total carbs) and subtract the 2g (dietary fiber).

- This will give us our net carbs of 4g.

Tips For Getting Started

Ketogenic dieting is a big jump for some people. You're switching over to a new metabolic substrate. That can take some getting used to. Make sure you are well-prepared with a Primalaligned eating pattern in place for ideally several weeks before you ponder a journey into nutritional ketosis.

Make a minimum commitment to six weeks of nutritional ketosis. You'll want to allow ample time for the transition to new fuel sources. Six weeks will put the metabolic machinery in place and allow you to begin experiencing the most dramatic benefits of keto living.

Get plenty of electrolytes. You'll want lots of sodium, magnesium, and potassium. Try 4.5 grams sodium (about two teaspoons of acceptable salt or a little under three teaspoons of kosher salt),

300-400mg magnesium, and 1- 2 grams of potassium each day on top of your regular food. Going keto flushes out water weight, and tons of electrolytes leave with it.

Eat extra fat during the first week to accelerate keto-adaptation. Just be sure to dial fat intake back after the first week or two.

Do lots of low-level aerobic activity. Walk, hike, jog, cycle, row. Keep things in the aerobic HR zone (under 180 minus age in heartbeats per minute), and you'll increase your utilization of body fat, which will speed up ketone production and adaptation.

Eat fiber. Many people on ketogenic diets tend to ignore fiber. That's a mistake. Fiber doesn't digest into glucose. It also supports your gut biome.

FASTING

Many studies have examined the benefits and risks of giving up food for a day, including how it affects weight loss. In this book, we look at what happens to the body during fasting and what a person can do to make fasting safer.

What happens during fasting?

Whether a person is fasting or not, the body still needs energy. Its primary energy source is a sugar called glucose, which usually comes from carbohydrates, including grains, dairy products, fruits, certain vegetables, beans, and even sweets.

The liver and muscles store the glucose and release it into the bloodstream whenever the body needs it. However, during fasting, this process changes. After about 8 hours of fasting, the liver will use the last of its glucose reserves. At this point, the body enters into a state called gluconeogenesis, marking the body's transition into fasting mode.

Studies have shown that gluconeogenesis increases the number of calories the body burns. With no carbohydrates coming in, the body creates its glucose using mainly fat. Eventually, the body runs out of these energy sources as well. Fasting mode then becomes the more serious starvation mode.

At this point, a person's metabolism slows down, and their body begins burning muscle tissue for energy.

Although it is a well-known term in dieting culture, the true starvation mode only occurs after several consecutive days or even weeks without food. So, for those breaking their fast after 24 hours, it is generally safe to go without eating for a day unless other health conditions are present.

Can fasting promote weight loss?

It does appear that fasting can help with weight loss. However, studies make it clear that this is not the case for everyone.

Popular diet plans include 12-hour or 16-hour fasting periods, as well as the 24-hour fast. Some diets require people to drink only water during the fast, while others allowed any zero-calorie beverage. Fasting is not necessarily better than any other weight-loss method, including reducing daily calorie intake by a small amount.

In a recent study, people with obesity who fasted intermittently for 12 months lost slightly more weight than those who dieted more traditionally, but the results were not statistically significant. The limits of fasting appear to have less to do with its physical effects than how it fits into a given lifestyle.

For example, the same study found that people who fasted were more likely to give up on weight-loss efforts than those who dieted in a more traditional way, such as counting calories. The researchers concluded that fasting might be harder to maintain over time.

Another possible concern is post-fast binging. Some fasting experts agree that it is easy to derail weight-loss successes by overeating after the fasting period. Fasting days can also offer a false sense of security, leading people to disregard positive eating habits on non-fasting days.

Other effects of fasting

As well as aiding weight loss, not eating for a day can have other health benefits. Research suggests that occasional 24-hour fasting can improve cardiovascular health. Some evidence from research on animals shows that fasting can help fight certain kinds of cancer or even help preserve memory.

Risks

Although it is generally safe, going a day without eating can be risky for some people, including:

- people with diabetes

- people with a history of eating disorders

- people using medications that they must take with food

- children and adolescents

- those who are pregnant or breastfeeding

WHAT IS THE SAFEST WAY TO BREAK A FAST?

According to Chelsey Amer, a registered dietitian nutritionist, there are several ways a person can break their fast safely:

Drink water: This is especially important if circumstances prevented it during the fast.

Eat a small meal: Eating a large meal immediately after a fast can strain the digestive system.

Chew food thoroughly: Chew each bite at least 30 times.

Eat cooked foods: Go for foods that are easier to digest, such as cooked vegetables instead of raw.

Avoid experimenting: Trying new foods after a fast can make digestion harder and make a person feel ill.

Summary

Going a day without eating is generally safe and can be beneficial in several ways, including a weight-loss tool. Fasting does not help weight loss any more than other conventional approaches and can be harder to stick with over the long term.

If a person is fasting for health reasons, they must do it safely and no longer than necessary. Long-term fasting starves the body of essential nutrients and can cause many complications.

"Fasting is not a weight loss tool. Fasting slows your metabolic rate down so your diet from before the fast is even more fattening after you fast," says Joel Fuhrman MD, author of Eat to Live: The Revolutionary Plan for Fast and Sustained Weight Loss and Fasting and Eating for Health.

Fasting for weight loss carries other health risks as well.

While fasting for a day or two is rarely a problem if you are healthy, "it can be quite dangerous if you are not already eating a healthy diet, or if you've got liver or kidney problems, any kind of compromised immune system functioning, or are on medication Even worse for dieters is that fasting for weight loss "distracts people from the real message of how to lose weight: lower fat intake, eat five fruits and vegetables a day, drink water and stop drinking other liquids, walk 30 minutes a day, and get more sleep," says Fernstrom, an associate professor of psychiatry, epidemiology, and surgery at the University of Pittsburgh School of Medicine.

Also, other practices that are often combined with fasting for weight loss, such as colon cleansing, carry their risks.

"Fasts are sometimes accompanied with enemas to cleanse your intestinal tract, and that can be very dangerous," says Fernstrom. "The intestinal tract has a lot of good bacteria. When you are changing that balance, the good bacteria are affected, too."

Here's where the debate gets intense. "There is no scientific evidence it will detox the body. The issue of fasting to cleanse the body has no biological basis because the body is real good at that by itself," says Fernstrom. "The liver is a natural detox center; the lungs, the colon, the kidneys, [the lymph glands] and the skin get rid of toxins."

"We know that the body is unable to rid itself of toxins when we eat a diet low in nutrients," and that applies to most Americans, even those who think they are healthy.

"Americans eat 51% of their diet from processed foods and foods low in phytochemicals and antioxidants," he says. "So you see a buildup of waste products in the cells -- AGE, advanced glycation end products -- that build up in cellular tissues and lead to atherosclerosis, aging, diabetes, nerve damage, and the deterioration of organs.

Along with improving your overall diet, fasting is one solution to that buildup of AGE, according to advocates. "Fasting allows the body to most effectively remove these waste products. The body is designed to fast; we do it every night."

How does fasting remove toxins from the body?

When you go without eating for more than a day or two, the body enters into ketosis. Ketosis occurs when the body runs out of carbohydrates to burn for energy, so it burns fat.

Medical Reasons for Fasting

Another topic on which there is medical agreement is the benefit - actually, the necessity -- of fasting before surgery. "You don't want the body to be digesting food as it manages the slower breathing [and other body changes] under anesthesia," says Fernstrom.

Fasting is also required to get accurate readings for certain medical tests. Short-term fasting before tests for cholesterol and blood sugar levels, for example, helps achieve a more accurate baseline count.

Fasting to Treat Disease

Fasting advocates also claim that the practice can effectively treat serious health conditions, from arthritis and colitis to heart disease and depression.

"Fasting followed by a vegetarian diet interferes with the immune system's activities, especially if the immune system is overreacting, as it does with ," and other auto-immune diseases, he says. He cites half a dozen studies published in medical journals ranging from the American Journal of Physiology-Endocrinology and Metabolism to the Scandinavian Journal of Rheumatology.

Studies published in The Proceedings of the National Academy of Sciences and The Journal of Nutrition in 2003 showed that mice forced to fast every other day, while eating twice the normal amount of food on non-fasting days, had better insulin control, neuronal resistance to injury, and other health indicators than mice fed calorie-restricted diets.

Fasting may yield psychological benefits as well. Use very brief fasting with my patients to help them cope with stress and depression.

Fasting for Longer Life

"There are hundreds of studies showing that when animals are fed fewer calories they live longer.

Studies on animals ranging from earthworms to monkeys have shown that alternating cycles of fasting and very calorie-restricted diets are a reliable way to extend the lifespan.

FASTING TIPS THAT'LL HELP YOU LOSE WEIGHT

Essentially, intermittent fasting (IF) is a type of eating plan that involves periods of fasting—during which you can consume only water, coffee, and tea—and eating—when you can generally eat what you like. Such freedom to choose your chow is one of the many reasons the diet's racked up so many fans, including stars like Vanessa Hudgens and Halle Berry.

And in a world where many of the top trending diets involve a lot of, well, math, IF stands out for being fairly simple to understand. "It doesn't require counting calories, macros, or measuring ketones. You can eat most anything you want between a specific window of time, although most programs recommend eating healthfully when you do eat.

Another pro? There isn't a one-size-fits-all plan or "right" way to do this, per Angelone. It's just the opposite. There are many different kinds of fasting, or IF schedules to choose from, so you can decide the diet that best fits your lifestyle. Here are a few popular picks:

The 16:8 diet: Eat whatever you want (read: no calorie counting!) for eight hours a day and fast for the rest.

The 5:2 diet: Eat normally for five days a week and cut back to 20 percent of your normal daily calories for the other two "fasting" days, which usually involves about 500 calories for women.

The 14:10 diet: Similar to the 16:8 method, but you fast only 14 hours and eat for 10, making it easier to follow but not necessarily easier to lose weight.

1. Ease into your new eating plan.

While it might be tempting to jump right into your new eating routine (the initial excitement is real), doing so can be difficult and leave you with increased hunger and discomfort, according to Michal Hertz, RD, a dietitian in New York City. Instead, she recommends starting slowly by, say, doing two to three days of IF during the first week and then "gradually increasing week to week." Taking thing slow isn't just a great fasting tip, but a great tip for life (just sayin').

2. Know the difference between needing to eat and wanting to eat.

Once you hear your stomach growl, it can feel like there's no way you'll get through X more amount of hours without food. Tune in to that hunger cue. "Ask yourself whether the hunger is boredom or actual hunger,

If you're truly hungry but not feeling weak or dizzy (which are signs, btw, that you should stop fasting ASAP), then sip a warm mint tea, as peppermint is known to reduce appetite, or drink water to help fill your stomach until your next meal, per Savage.

Now, if you've been trying IF for a while and still feel extreme hunger between periods, then you need to do some thinking. "You need to either add more nutrient- or calorie-dense foods during your eight-hour period, or consider that this may not be the best plan for you," Hertz says. Adding healthy fats such as nut butter, avocado, and coconut and olive oils, as well as proteins, during eating times can help keep you stay satisfied and full longer.

3. Eat when necessary.

Technically, intense hunger and fatigue shouldn't happen when following the 16:8 fasting method (perhaps the most common one). But if you feel extremely lightheaded, listen up, as odds are your body's trying to tell you something. You likely have low blood sugar and need to eat something—and repeat after me, that is okay.

By definition, fasting involves removing some, if not all, food, so don't beat yourself up for breaking your fast with small—and smart!—bites. Your best bet? Go for a protein-rich snack like a few slices of turkey breast or one to two hard-boiled eggs (to help remain in a ketogenic (fat-burning) state), Savage recommends. You can then return fasting, that is, of course, if you feel up to it.

4. Hydrate, hydrate, hydrate.

Even when you're fasting, drinking water and bevies like coffee and tea (sans milk) are not just allowed, but, especially in the case of H2O, encouraged. Setting reminders throughout the day and particularly during fasting periods to lap up plenty of liquids. Aim to fill up on at least 2, if not 3, liters per day, according to both Hertz and Savage.

5. Break your fast slowly and steadily.

After spending several hours food-free, you might feel like a human vacuum ready to suck up whatever's on your plate. But chowing down in minutes is no Bueno for your body or your waistline, according to research. Instead, you want to chew well and eat slowly to allow your digestive system to fully process the food, Savage explains. This will also help you have a better idea of your fullness so that you steer clear of overeating.

6. Avoid overeating.

On that note, just because you've stopped fasting doesn't mean you should feast. Not only can eating too much leave you bloated and uncomfortable, but it can also sabotage the weight-loss goals that likely led you to IF in the first place. Simply put: It's not necessarily how much is on your plate that can help you stay full for longer but what is on your plate. This brings me to the next fasting tip...

7. Maintain balanced meals.

Having a hearty mixture of protein, fiber, healthy fats, and carbs can help you ultimately shed those pounds and steer clear of extreme hunger when fasting. A good example, per Savage? Grilled chicken (you want about 4 to 6 oz of protein) with half of a small sweet potato, and sautéed spinach with garlic and olive oil.

When it comes to fruits, you want to opt for those with "a low-glycemic index, which are more slowly digested, absorbed, and metabolized, causing a lower and slower rise in blood glucose. A stable blood-sugar level helps you avoid cravings—and thus is key when it comes to successfully dropping lbs.

8. Play around with different periods.

Look at your general lifestyle to see which fasting method might fit best. For example, if you're an early riser, eating during the earlier hours, like 10 am to 6 pm, and then fasting until the following morning at 10. Remember: The beauty of IF is that it's easily amendable and flexible to fit you and your schedule.

According to Savage, another option is cutting yourself off earlier and eating breakfast later each day to gradually grow your fasting strength. "We all naturally fast once daily—while we sleep—so maybe you practice 'shutting down the kitchen' earlier." For example, "close" the kitchen at 9 pm, and then don't eat again until breakfast at 8 am. That's a natural 11-hour fast! Slowly move those times out (e.g., kitchen closes at 8 pm, breakfast at 9 am),

Adapt your workout routine.

First thing's first: You can most definitely exercise if you're doing a fasting diet. But (!!) you want to be mindful of what types of movement you do, and when. "If you're choosing to exercise in a fasting state, I would recommend exercising first thing in the morning, when you may have the most energy, it's important to remember that if you're not, in Savage's words, "adequately fueling your muscles," then you're at a greater risk of injury. So you might want to consider lower-impact workouts, such as yoga or steady-state cardio, on fasting mornings and save that hard-core HIIT class for after you've eaten.

11. Keep track of your journey.

Believe it or not, maintaining a food journal can help you with your fasting diet. A food journal for fasting?! Yup, you read that right. While you might not be chronicling as many eats, actively jotting down details like any emotions and symptoms (hunger level, any weakness, etc.) that come up during IF can help you gauge your progress, Savage says. (It might also help you notice any trigger points that make fasting harder on you, like drinking the night prior.)

12. Listen to your body.

This. Is. Important. Keep an eye out at all times for symptoms such as dizziness, fatigue, (unusual) irritability, headache, anxiety, and difficulty concentrating. If you experience any of these, consider breaking your fast. "These are all signs that the body is going into starvation mode and may need nourishment," Savage says. And if you start to feel colder than normal, that is even more of a sign to stop fasting, she adds.

That said, be patient. It'll likely take your body time to get used to fasting, and you may feel hungrier and weaker than usual. So don't flip out if you have these (less serious) sensations for a week or so. However, if these challenges last longer and you experience symptoms like the ones above dizziness, Savage recommends ditching the diet and finding something else to help you meet your goals. No amount of pounds is worth getting sick over—trust.

WEIGHT LOSS

What's the best diet for healthy weight loss?

Pick up any diet book, and it will claim to hold all the answers to successfully losing all the weight you want—and keeping it off. Some claim the key is to eat less and exercise more, others that low fat is the only way to go, while others prescribe cutting out carbs. So, what should you believe? The truth is there is no "one size fits all" solution to permanent healthy weight loss. What works for one person may not work for you since our bodies respond differently to different foods, depending on genetics and other health factors. To find the method of weight loss that's right for you will likely take time and require patience, commitment, and some experimentation with different foods and diets.

While some people respond well to counting calories or similar restrictive methods, others respond better to having more freedom in planning their weight-loss programs. Being free to avoid fried foods or cut back on refined carbs can set them up for success. So, don't get too discouraged if a diet that worked for somebody else doesn't work for you. And don't beat yourself up if a diet proves too restrictive for you to stick with. Ultimately, a diet is only right for you if it's one you can stick with over time.

Remember: while there's no easy fix to losing weight, there are plenty of steps you can take to develop a healthier relationship with food, curb emotional triggers to overeating, and achieve a healthy weight.

Cut calories some experts believe that successfully managing your weight comes down to a simple equation: If you eat fewer calories than you burn, you lose weight. Sounds easy, right? Then why is losing weight so hard?

·   Weight loss isn't a linear event over time. When you cut calories, you may drop weight for the first few weeks, for example, and then something changes. You eat the same number of calories, but you lose less weight or no weight at all. That's because when you lose weight, you're losing water and lean tissue as well as fat, your metabolism slows, and your body changes in other ways. So, to continue dropping weight each week, you need to continue cutting calories.

·   A calorie isn't always a calorie. Eating 100 calories of high fructose corn syrup, for example, can have a different effect on your body than eating 100 calories of broccoli. The trick for sustained weight loss is to ditch the foods packed with calories but don't make you feel full (like candy) and replace them with foods that fill you up without being loaded with calories (like vegetables).

·   Many of us don't always eat simply to satisfy hunger. We also turn to food for comfort or relieve stress—which can quickly derail any weight loss plan.

1. Cut carbs

A different way of viewing weight loss identifies the problem as consuming too many calories, but rather the way the body accumulates fat after consuming carbohydrates—in particular, the role of the hormone insulin. When you eat a meal, carbohydrates from the food enter your bloodstream as glucose. To keep your blood sugar levels in check, your body always burns off this glucose before it burns off fat from a meal.

If you eat a carbohydrate-rich meal (lots of pasta, rice, bread, or French fries, for example), your body releases insulin to help with the influx of all this glucose into your blood. As well as regulating blood sugar levels, insulin does two things: It prevents your fat cells from releasing fat for the body to burn as fuel (because its priority is to burn off the glucose), and it creates more fat cells for storing everything that your body can't burn off.

The result is that you gain weight and your body now requires more fuel to burn, so you eat more. Since insulin only burns carbohydrates, you crave carbs, and so begins a vicious cycle of consuming carbs and gaining weight. To lose weight, the reasoning goes, you need to break this cycle by reducing carbs.

Most low-carb diets advocate replacing carbs with protein and fat, which could have some negative long-term effects on your health. If you try a low-carb diet, you can reduce your risks and limit your intake of saturated and trans fats by choosing lean meats, fish and vegetarian sources of protein, low-fat dairy products, and eating plenty of leafy green and non-starchy vegetables.

1. Cut fat

It's a mainstay of many diets: if you don't want to get fat, don't eat fat. Walk down any grocery store aisle, and you'll be bombarded with reduced-fat snacks, dairy, and packaged meals. But while our low-fat options have exploded, so have obesity rates. So, why haven't low-fat diets worked for more of us?

1. Not all fat is bad. Healthy or "good" fats can help control your weight and manage your moods and fight fatigue. Unsaturated fats found in avocados, nuts, seeds, soy milk, tofu, and fatty fish can help fill you up, while adding a little tasty olive oil to a plate of vegetables, for example, can make it easier to eat healthy food and improve the overall quality of your diet.

2. We often make the wrong trade-offs. Many of us make the mistake of swapping fat for the empty calories of sugar and refined carbohydrates. Instead of eating whole-fat yogurt, for example, we eat low- or no-fat versions packed with sugar to make up for the loss of taste. Or we swap our fatty breakfast bacon for a muffin or donut that causes rapid spikes in blood sugar.

1. Follow the Mediterranean diet.

The Mediterranean diet emphasizes eating good fats and good carbs along with large quantities of fresh fruits and vegetables, nuts, fish, and olive oil—and only modest amounts of meat and cheese. The Mediterranean diet is more than just about food, though. Regular physical activity and sharing meals with others are also major components.

Whatever weight-loss strategy you try, it's important to stay motivated and avoid common dieting pitfalls, such as emotional eating.

Control emotional eating

We don't always eat simply to satisfy hunger. All too often, we turn to food when we're stressed or anxious, which can wreck any diet and pack on the pounds. Do you eat when you're worried, bored, or lonely? Do you snack in front of the TV at the end of a stressful day? Recognizing your emotional eating triggers can make all the difference in your weight-loss efforts. If you eat when you're:

Stressed – find healthier ways to calm yourself. Try yoga, meditation, or soaking in a hot bath.

Low on energy – find other mid-afternoon pick-me-ups. Try walking around the block, listening to energizing music, or taking a short nap.

Lonely or bored – reach out to others instead of reaching for the refrigerator. Call a friend who makes you laugh, take your dog for a walk, or go to the library, mall, or park—anywhere there are people.

Practice mindful eating instead

- Avoid distractions while eating. Try not to eat while working, watching TV, or driving. It's too easy to mindlessly overeat.

- Pay attention. Eat slowly, savoring the smells and textures of your food. If your mind wanders, gently return your attention to your food and how it tastes.

- Mix things up to focus on the experience of eating. Try using chopsticks rather than a fork, or use your utensils with your non-dominant hand.

- Stop eating before you are full. It takes time for the signal to reach your brain that you've had enough. Don't feel obligated to always clean your plate.

Stay motivated

Permanent weight loss requires making healthy changes to your lifestyle and food choices. To stay motivated:

Find a cheering section. Social support means a lot. Programs like Jenny Craig and Weight Watchers use group support to impact weight loss and lifelong healthy eating. Seek out support—whether in the form of family, friends, or a support group—to get the encouragement you need. Slow and steady wins the race. Losing weight too fast can take a toll on your mind and body, making you feel sluggish, drained, and sick. Aim to lose one to two pounds a week, so you're losing fat rather than water and muscle.

Set goals to keep you motivated. Short-term goals, like wanting to fit into a bikini for the summer, usually don't work as well as wanting to feel more confident or become healthier for your children's sakes. When temptation strikes, focus on the benefits you'll reap from being healthier.
Use tools to track your progress. Smartphone apps, fitness trackers, or simply keeping a journal can help you keep track of the food you eat, the calories you burn, and the weight you lose. Seeing the results in black and white can help you stay motivated.

Get plenty of sleep. Lack of sleep stimulates your appetite, so you want more food than normal; at the same time, it stops you from feeling satisfied, making you want to keep eating. Sleep deprivation can also affect your motivation, so aim for eight hours of quality sleep a night.

Cut down on sugar and refined carbs.

Whether or not you're specifically aiming to cut carbs, most of us consume unhealthy amounts of sugar and refined carbohydrates such as white bread, pizza dough, pasta, pastries, white flour, white rice, and sweetened breakfast cereals. Replacing refined carbs with their whole-grain counterparts and eliminating candy and desserts is only part of the solution, though. Sugar is hidden in foods as diverse as canned soups and vegetables, pasta sauce, margarine, and many reduced fat foods. Since your body gets all it needs from sugar naturally occurring in food, all this added sugar amounts to nothing but many empty calories and unhealthy spikes in your blood glucose.

Less sugar can mean a slimmer waistline.

Calories obtained from fructose (found in sugary beverages such as soda and processed foods like doughnuts, muffins, and candy) are more likely to add to fat around your belly. Cutting back on sugary foods can mean a slimmer waistline as well as a lower risk of diabetes.

Fill up with fruit, veggies, and fiber.

Even if you're cutting calories, that doesn't necessarily mean you have to eat less food. High-fiber foods such as fruit, vegetables, beans, and whole grains are higher in volume and take longer to digest, making them filling—and great for weight-loss.

- It's generally okay to eat as much fresh fruit and non-starchy vegetables as you want— you'll feel full before you've overdone it on the calories.

- Eat vegetables raw or steamed, not fried or breaded, and dress them with herbs and spices or a little olive oil for flavor.

- Add fruit to low sugar cereal—blueberries, strawberries, sliced bananas. You'll still enjoy lots of sweetness, but with fewer calories, less sugar, and more fiber.

- Bulk out sandwiches by adding healthy veggie choices like lettuce, tomatoes, sprouts, cucumbers, and avocado.

- Snack on carrots or celery with hummus instead of high-calorie chips and dip.

- Add more veggies to your favorite main courses to make your dish more substantial. Even pasta and stir-fries can be diet-friendly if you use fewer noodles and more vegetables.

- Start your meal with salad or vegetable soup to help fill you up, so you eat less of your entrée.

- Take charge of your food environment.

- Set yourself up for weight-loss success by taking charge of your food environment: when you eat, how much you eat, and what foods you make easily available.

- Cook your meals at home. This allows you to control both portion size and what goes into the food. Restaurant and packaged foods generally contain a lot more sugar, unhealthy fat, and calories than food cooked at home—plus the portion sizes tend to be larger.

- Serve yourself smaller portions. Use small plates, bowls, and cups to make your portions appear larger. Don't eat out of large bowls or directly from food containers, making it difficult to assess how much you've eaten.

- Eat early. Studies suggest that consuming more of your daily calories at breakfast and fewer at dinner can help you drop more pounds. Eating a larger, healthy breakfast can jump-start your metabolism, stop you from feeling hungry during the day, and give you more time to burn off the calories.

- Fast for 14 hours a day. Try to eat dinner earlier in the day and then fast until breakfast the next morning. Eating only when you're most active and giving your digestion a long break may aid in weight loss.

- Plan your meals and snacks ahead of time. You can create your small portion snacks in plastic bags or containers. Eating on a schedule will help you avoid eating when you aren't truly hungry.

- Drink more water. Thirst can often be confused with hunger, so by drinking water, you can avoid extra calories.

- Limit the number of tempting foods you have at home. If you share a kitchen with non-dieters, store indulgent foods out of sight.

Get moving

The degree to which exercise aids weight loss is open to debate, but the benefits go way beyond burning calories. Exercise can increase your metabolism and improve your outlook—and it's something you can benefit from right now. Go for a walk, stretch, move around, and you'll have more energy and motivation to tackle the other steps in your weight-loss program.

Lack time for a long workout? Three 10-minute spurts of exercise per day can be just as good as one 30-minute workout.

Remember: anything is better than nothing. Start slowly with small amounts of physical activity each day. Then, as you start to lose weight and have more energy, you'll find it easier to become more physically active.

Find an exercise you enjoy. Try walking with a friend, dancing, hiking, cycling, playing Frisbee with a dog, enjoying a pickup game of basketball, or playing activity-based video games with your kids.

Keeping the weight off

You may have heard the widely quoted statistic that 95% of people who lose weight on a diet will regain it within a few years—or even months. While there isn't much hard evidence to support that claim, many weight-loss plans indeed fail in the long term. Often that's simply because diets that are too restrictive are very hard to maintain over time. However, that doesn't mean your weight loss attempts are doomed to failure, far from it.

INTERMITTENT FASTING

What Is Intermittent Fasting (IF)?

Intermittent fasting (IF) is an eating pattern that cycles between periods of fasting and eating. It doesn't specify which foods you should eat but rather when you should eat them. In this respect, it's not a diet in the conventional sense but more accurately described as an eating pattern. Common intermittent fasting methods involve daily 16-hour fasts or fasting for 24 hours, twice per week.

Fasting has been a practice throughout human evolution. Ancient hunter-gatherers didn't have supermarkets, refrigerators, or food available year-round. Sometimes they couldn't find anything to eat. As a result, humans evolved to be able to function without food for extended periods. Fasting from time to time is more natural than always eating 3–4 (or more) meals per day.

Summary

Intermittent fasting (IF) is an eating pattern that cycles between periods of fasting and eating. It's currently very popular in the health and fitness community.

Intermittent Fasting Methods

There are several different ways of doing intermittent fasting — all of which involve splitting the day or week into eating and fasting periods.

During the fasting periods, you eat either very little or nothing at all.

These are the most popular methods:

The 16/8 method: Also called the Leangains protocol, it involves skipping breakfast and restricting your daily eating period to 8 hours, such as 1–9 pm. Then you fast for 16 hours in between.

Eat-Stop-Eat: This involves fasting for 24 hours, once or twice a week, for example, by not eating from dinner one day until dinner the next day.

The 5:2 diet: With this method, you consume only 500–600 calories on two non-consecutive days of the week but normally eat the other five days.

All of these methods should cause weight loss by reducing your calorie intake as long as you don't compensate by eating much more during the eating periods. Many people find the 16/8 method the simplest, most sustainable, and easiest to stick to. It's also the most popular.

Summary

There are several different ways to do intermittent fasting. All of them split the day or week into eating and fasting periods.

- When you fast, several things happen in your body on the cellular and molecular level.

- For example, your body adjusts hormone levels to make stored body fat more accessible.

- Your cells also initiate important repair processes and change the expression of genes.

Here are some changes that occur in your body when you fast:

Human Growth Hormone (HGH): The growth hormone levels skyrocket, increasing as much as 5-fold. This has benefits for fat loss and muscle gain, to name a few.

Insulin: Insulin sensitivity improves, and levels of insulin drop dramatically. Lower insulin levels make stored body fat more accessible.

Cellular repair: When fasted, your cells initiate cellular repair processes. This includes autophagy, where cells digest and remove old and dysfunctional proteins that build up inside cells.

Gene expression: There are changes in the function of genes related to longevity and protection against disease.

These changes in hormone levels, cell function, and gene expression are responsible for the health benefits of intermittent fasting.

Summary

When you fast, human growth hormone levels go up, and insulin levels go down. Your body's cells also change the expression of genes and initiate important cellular repair processes.

A Very Powerful Weight Loss Tool

- Weight loss is the most common reason for people to try intermittent fasting.

- By making you eat fewer meals, intermittent fasting can lead to an automatic reduction in calorie intake.

- Additionally, intermittent fasting changes hormone levels to facilitate weight loss.

- In addition to lowering insulin and increasing growth hormone levels, it increases the fat-burning hormone norepinephrine (noradrenaline).

- Because of these changes in hormones, short-term fasting may increase your metabolic rate by 3.6–14%.

- By helping you eat fewer and burn more calories, intermittent fasting causes weight loss by changing both calorie equation sides.

- Studies show that intermittent fasting can be a very powerful weight-loss tool.

- A 2014 review study found that this eating pattern can cause 3–8% weight loss over 3–24 weeks, which is a significant amount compared to most weight loss studies.

- According to the same study, people also lost 4–7% of their waist circumference, indicating a significant loss of harmful belly fat that builds up around your organs and causes disease.

- Another study showed that intermittent fasting causes less muscle loss than the more standard continuous calorie restriction.

- However, keep in mind that the main reason for its success is that intermittent fasting helps you eat fewer calories overall. If you binge and eat massive amounts during your eating periods, you may not lose any weight at all.

Summary

Intermittent fasting may slightly boost metabolism while helping you eat fewer calories. It's a very effective way to lose weight and belly fat.

HEALTH BENEFITS

Many studies have been done on intermittent fasting in both animals and humans. These studies have shown that it can have powerful benefits for weight control and your body and brain's health. It may even help you live longer.

Here are the main health benefits of intermittent fasting:

Weight loss: As mentioned above, intermittent fasting can help you lose weight and belly fat without consciously restricting calories.

Insulin resistance: Intermittent fasting can reduce insulin resistance, lowering blood sugar by 3–6% and fasting insulin levels by 20–31%, which should protect against type 2 diabetes.

Inflammation: Some studies show reductions in markers of inflammation, a key driver of many chronic diseases.

Heart health: Intermittent fasting may reduce "bad" LDL cholesterol, blood triglycerides, inflammatory markers, blood sugar, and insulin resistance — all risk factors for heart disease.

Cancer: Animal studies suggest that intermittent fasting may prevent cancer.

Brain health: Intermittent fasting increases the brain hormone BDNF and may aid new nerve cells' growth. It may also protect against Alzheimer's disease.

Anti-aging: Intermittent fasting can extend lifespan in rats. Studies showed that fasted rats lived 36–83% longer.

Keep in mind that research is still in its early stages. Many of the studies were small, short-term, or conducted in animals. Many questions have yet to be answered in higher quality human studies.

Summary

Intermittent fasting can have many benefits for your body and brain. It can cause weight loss and reduce your risk of type 2 diabetes, heart disease, and cancer. It may also help you live longer.

Makes Your Healthy Lifestyle Simpler

- Eating healthy is simple, but it can be incredibly hard to maintain. One of the main obstacles is all the work required to plan for and cook healthy meals.

- Intermittent fasting can make things easier, as you don't need to plan, cook or clean up after as many meals as before.

- For this reason, intermittent fasting is very popular among the life-hacking crowd, as it improves your health while simplifying your life at the same time.

Summary

One of the major benefits of intermittent fasting is that it makes healthy eating simpler. There are fewer meals you need to prepare, cook and clean up after.

Who Should Be Careful Or Avoid It?

Intermittent fasting is certainly not for everyone. If you're underweight or have a history of eating disorders, you should not fast without consulting with a health professional first. In these cases, it can be downright harmful.

Should Women Fast?

- There is some evidence that intermittent fasting may not be as beneficial for women as men. For example, one study showed that it improved insulin sensitivity in men but worsened blood sugar control in women.

- Though human studies on this topic are unavailable, studies in rats have found that intermittent fasting can make female rats emaciated, masculinized, infertile, and cause them to miss cycles.

- Several anecdotal reports of women whose menstrual period stopped when they started doing IF and went back to normal when they resumed their previous eating pattern.

- For these reasons, women should be careful with intermittent fasting.

- They should follow separate guidelines, like easing into the practice and stopping immediately if they have any problems like amenorrhea (absence of menstruation).

- If you have fertility issues and are trying to conceive, consider holding off on intermittent fasting for now. This eating pattern is likely also a bad idea if you're pregnant or breastfeeding.

Summary

People who are underweight or have a history of eating disorders should not fast. There is also some evidence that intermittent fasting may be harmful to some women.

Safety and Side Effects

- Hunger is the main side effect of intermittent fasting.

- You may also feel weak, and your brain may not perform as well as you're used to.

- This may only be temporary, as it can take some time for your body to adapt to the new meal schedule.

- If you have a medical condition, you should consult with your doctor before trying intermittent fasting.

This is particularly important if you:

- Have diabetes.

- Have problems with blood sugar regulation.

- Have low blood pressure.

- Take medications.

- Are underweight.

- Have a history of eating disorders.

- Are a woman who is trying to conceive.

- Are a woman with a history of amenorrhea.

- Are you pregnant or breastfeeding?

All that being said, intermittent fasting has an outstanding safety profile. There is nothing dangerous about not eating for a while if you're healthy and well-nourished overall.

Summary

The most common side effect of intermittent fasting is hunger. People with certain medical conditions should not fast without consulting with a doctor first.